He  Antibiotics and Antivirals:

Herbal Medicine to Heal Yourself Naturally

By

Brittany Samons

Table of Contents

Introduction 5

Chapter 1. Antibiotic and The Rise of Superbugs 7

Chapter 2. Herbal Antibiotics: Nature's Arsenal Against Superbugs 11

Chapter 3. Benefits of Using Herbal Antibiotics and Antivirals 16

Chapter 4. Common Preparation Methods for Antibacterial and Antiviral Herbs 19

Chapter 5. Foods and Herbs That Have Antibacterial and Antiviral Properties 22

Chapter 6. Role of Immune System 29

Conclusion 32

Thank You Page 33

Herbal Antibiotics and Antivirals: Herbal Medicine to Heal Yourself Naturally

By Brittany Samons

© Copyright 2015 Brittany Samons

Reproduction or translation of any part of this work beyond that permitted by section 107 or 108 of the 1976 United States Copyright Act without permission of the copyright owner is unlawful. Requests for permission or further information should be addressed to the author.

This publication is designed to provide accurate and authoritative information in regard to the subject matter covered. This work is sold with the understanding that the publisher is not engaged in rendering legal, accounting, or other professional services. If legal advice or other expert assistance is required, the services of a competent professional person should be sought.

First Published, 2015

Printed in the United States of America

Introduction

Every day, as more and more people use antibiotics, new stronger strains of bacteria are produced. The downside of this is that there will come a time when nothing created from the laboratory will even react with bacteria due to the degree of resistance the bacteria have already acquired.

One of the most undesirable effects of antibiotics is that they disable the immune system. This is detrimental since other microorganisms and viruses, which lay dormant or are kept at bay by the immune system, could have a chance of populating or affecting the body.

Herbal antibiotics are nature's arsenal against microorganism. Plants have evolved to produce chemical compounds with the intent of killing both bacteria and viruses to protect itself against their attacks. Thus, their chemical makeup is fit to kill without giving the bacteria the chance of adapting to it.

The era of the antibiotics is its inevitable end. Bacteria are already gaining pace against it. The fight against infectious diseases turns anew. This time, nature is with us in this fight.

Contained in this book are detailed information about the antiviral and antibacterial properties of herbs along with the detailed account of how these properties enable them to kill these microorganisms. There is a list of herbs to choose from with regard to their potencies, how they are used, what they treat and the preparation method most appropriate. The preparation methods used for herbs are also included.

Chapter 1. Antibiotic and The Rise of Superbugs

When antibiotics were discovered in 1928, it was thought of that time that the fight for infectious diseases ends and that the word entered a new era of empowered resistance against the attack of bacteria.

Since the initial discovery of antibiotics, more than 100 types and variants were discovered. Since there is no other means to combat deadly bacterial attacks, many have relied on these medicines.

By 1999, however, 54 years after it was produced for commercial purposes, the miracle drug began showing signs of failure and inability to cure diseases, and the first three victims fell prey to the first superbug—a breed of new bacteria that are resistant to all available antibiotics at that time. Today, superbugs abound throughout the world's population.

When Bugs Turn Super

Bacteria are among the organisms on the earth that can reproduce at a fast rate. A generation can be replaced by another in a mere 20 minutes. Because of this, bacteria are among the organisms who have the most excellent methods of adaptation at the genetic level. At certain moments, one or few of a culture of bacteria exposed to an antibiotic will develop resistance. This resistance can be transferred to other bacteria rendering them as resistant as well. This process could continue against other forms of antibiotics. Eventually, a culture of bacteria able to resist all clinical forms of antibiotics is produced. These bacteria, also known as multidrug resistant (MDR) bacteria, are what we call superbugs.

There are two ways that bacteria can develop resistance to antibiotics:

1. Mutation in the DNA of the bacteria

Often, antibiotics work by deactivating a bacterial protein necessary for it to function normally. Genetic mutations within the DNA of bacteria can make it operate without that protein by altogether removing it. Another way of resistance is the production of a protein with a different structure thereby preventing antibiotics to attach to it or subsequently deactivate it. Genetic mutation can also enable the increased production of the abovementioned protein or enzyme thereby rendering the antibiotic unable to deactivate all the proteins. Bacteria could also develop the propensity to produce compounds or enzymes that are capable of deactivating the antibiotics. Lastly, genetic mutation can cause a difference in the permeability of its cell wall (or the capacity to allow and disallow the passage of substances via the cell membrane) thereby preventing the entry of antibiotics.

2. Transfer of the antibiotic genes from one bacterium to other bacteria

This is similar to sharing safety guidelines from a bacterium to another only that they are sent through a DNA section that each bacterium could copy.

The Fight against Bacteria Goes On

Until a new class of compounds that are able to disarm or disable bacteria in a different way is discovered, antibiotics will remain to be one of our most potent weapons against these microorganisms. The resistance a bacterium develops is also linked. That means the resistance bacteria develop against an antibiotic will work on other antibiotics as well. Bacteria can lose the resistance they gain against antibiotics but only under certain rare conditions. Furthermore, this mechanism is not always simple and easy. It is safe to assume, however, that when antibiotic therapies are limited, superbugs are less likely to develop.

There is an alternative, however, to this costly and superbugs-producing medication—taking advantage of the natural antibacterial arsenals of nature in the form of herbal medicine. The compounds that are naturally found in some plants are capable of killing bacteria without giving them the chance to develop resistance.

Chapter 2. Herbal Antibiotics: Nature's Arsenal Against Superbugs

Under normal conditions, our body is fully capable of defending itself against microorganisms. However, bacteria and viruses develop certain adaptation mechanisms in order to survive the harsh environment inside our bodies. Most of these bacteria (and viruses) are either dormant, beneficial (in the case of gut bacteria) or harmless. A percentage of bacteria, however, produces toxic substances and are harmful to our body.

During the discovery of penicillin, the world believed that a drug capable of shutting off bacterial activity and giving solution to infectious diseases has been developed. Little did they know that the success was short-lived and that the careless use of it has caused the mutation of bacteria into superbugs.

Herbal medicine, being naturally occurring and is designed by nature to purposely defend the plant against bacterial (or viral, in some cases) attacks, are different. Although the action of different classes of antibiotics differs from one type of bacteria to another, their mechanism of action is somewhat similar in a way. This mechanism of action is classified by experts as simple and that bacteria are capable of surviving them by developing simple resistance mechanisms.

Herbal compounds, however, are different. Each plant has a characteristic mechanism of action against microorganism. Furthermore, their chemical compositions are sometimes complex making it difficult for the bacteria to create a defense mechanism against those.

Three Types of Herbal Antibiotics

There is a wide range of plants and a number of plant-derived compounds that are capable of arresting bacterial activity through a number of functions.

Here a list of the three types of herbal antibiotics:

1) Systemic antibacterials – these are plant-based and plant-derived compounds that are consumed or introduced into the bloodstream and circulate throughout the body to each cell and organ to perform its action. They are best used to treat resistant infections that spread throughout the entire system.

2) Localized antibacterials – these compounds or herbal products do not circulate throughout the body in contrast to systemic antibacterials. Their effect is limited to one side or a small area and is good against infections in the skin and urinary and gastrointestinal tracks. They are either applied locally to stop bacterial infection on the skin or ingested to address infections of the GI tracks (such as E. coli, cholera or o157:H7) or of the urinary track.

3) Facilitative herbs – also called synergistic herbs, these are herbs that potentiates the action of other herbal or pharmaceutical products or substances. They weaken the bacteria by disabling their antibiotic-neutralizing actions, improve the body's performance to assist in combating the bacteria or potentiate a function of another substance.

Combining Plants for More Antibacterial Power

Compounds from plants are highly complex being nature's powerful chemical factories. Thus, plant-derived antibacterials are extremely dangerous to bacterial life. When taken into combinations, however, especially in synergistic mixtures, their potencies and effects are greatly enhanced.

Furthermore, mixing plants during medicinal preparations increase the solubility and reduce or neutralize the irritating effects of some plants.

Systemic Herbal Antibiotics

A significant number of diseases, like those caused by Staphylococcus bacteria, spread throughout the body and are manifested through various forms. They are able to reach internal organs and parts of the body that cannot be easily accessed. In order to address staphylococcus-related diseases, a systemic herbal antibiotic must be used.

Systemic herbal antibiotic spread throughout the body and arrest bacterial activity and growth wherever they are located.

The problem with resistant forms of bacterial infection is that, once you are afflicted by it and once every form of antibiotic medication does not have any effects on it anymore, there would be no other option aside from herbal medications. The good thing about herbal antibacterial medications is that they are able to affect bacteria even those that already acquired resistance.

When taken orally, herbs that have antibacterial properties and the compounds responsible for the said property are stored in the intestinal membranes and are delivered to various parts of the body such as the kidneys and the liver. Some are systemic—they enter the bloodstream; are widely circulated; reach almost every cell within the body and are concentrated on various areas such as the liver. Examples of this are the herbs and plants used to cure malaria. Although there are herbs that only address the symptoms of the disease (and which should be analyzed and avoided, if necessary), the antibacterial types are capable of killing the bacteria in the body.

Chapter 3. Benefits of Using Herbal Antibiotics and Antivirals

Herbs are known to be sources of natural antibacterial compounds, which our body are able to tolerate. The following benefits make herbal antibiotics preferable to pharmaceutical ones:

Cost less. The more potent the antibiotic is, the more expensive it gets. Often, the last line classes of antibiotics prescribed for infectious diseases that no longer respond to medication are the costliest. Herbs, on the other are cheaper. Since bacteria do not develop resistance against it, there is no need of consuming preparations with higher concentration at a higher price. They can even be grown at home in order to ensure a fresh and free supply of these plants and herbs.

Do not produce superbugs. Unlike antibiotics which bacteria develop resistance for, herbs are complex and affect bacteria in a more lethal and effective way, thus, not giving them time to develop resistance. Because of this, the same dosage and type of herb can be administered in the future should a similar infection occur without decrease in its potency, its effects or its ability to bring about cure.

Are easy to prepare. Herbal preparations do not require the costly and controlled processes pharmaceutical antibiotics undergo. They can be prepared at home with the use of simple tools and are easy to store, as well, for future use.

Are ecologically friendly. Planting herbs for future use benefit the earth. This is an activity that you can do in excess without bad effects.

Are potent and effective. The compounds plant use could cleave the DNA of bacteria, viruses (and even cancer cells). In addition, each herb has unique qualities that add up to make a more holistic and effective arsenal against bacteria.

Have nourishing effects. When pharmaceutical antibiotics are used to treat an infection, it interferes with the mechanisms within the body. They are also difficult to remove from the system and have hosts of side effects. In comparison, herbal antibiotics are not ingested or used as a pure substance but rather as a simple preparation. These preparations, often including roots, leaves and stems and other plant parts, retain other beneficial compounds they contain such as antioxidants, vitamins, minerals, healing factors and anti-inflammatories. Thus, instead of producing negative side effects, they produce a host of other beneficial effects to the body, as well, assisting it in the recovery phase after the bacteria have been neutralized.

Chapter 4. Common Preparation Methods for Antibacterial and Antiviral Herbs

Although it will take a significant portion of your time, preparing your own herbal medicine will not only save you money but will also assure you of the quality of your preparations. Here are the common preparation methods for antibacterial and antiviral herbs:

Infusions. This method of preparation is used for more sensitive herbs and plant parts such as leaves and tender plants. The preparation is similar to tea making: you pour a hot boiling water over fresh herbs and you let it sit for about 10-15 minutes. Another way of doing this is to drop plant parts to a pot of boiling water and allow it to steep for a while. The infusion is then filtered and kept or consumed. Other infusion methods include using alcohol and oil as a solvent instead of hot water. You allow the plant part to sit in an alcohol and oil for days or months or until the substance in the plant dissolves in the solvent.

Decoction. For the tougher plant parts where infusion might not dissolve all necessary compounds, decoction is more necessary. Instead of letting it sit to hot water, plant parts such as stem, bark, roots or seeds are boiled in water for a longer period of time until the material softens or until the active substances in it are dissolved.

Strong decoction. A more robust form of allowing its active constituents to dissolve is used with harder plant material that cannot be processed with just boiling them down for few minutes. Strong decoction is performed by either boiling the plant part longer (usually for hours on end) or by boiling them above the boiling point (with the use of pressure cooking pots) and allowing them to soak in the water overnight or for several days. When straining, the plant parts are further pressed intensely to extract whatever extractable fluids remain.

Tinctures. When compounds from the herb are not soluble (or readily soluble) to water, this method of preparation is used. This method requires that the plant material is placed in a container with a 40% spirit of ethanol (or methanol) or more is added. The mixture is then left for half a month to three weeks and is shaken at times to facilitate the transfer of active ingredients in the plants to the solvent.

Maceration. In this preparation, the leaves or the more tender parts of an herb are added to a liquid and allowed to soak for 12-24 hours. The liquid is the recovered and used. Another method is to add in ground powder forms of plants into water juice or beverage and consume.

Percolation. In this method, the plant material is placed above a filter, and a hot water is made to pass through it. The water that drains is then collected for consumption or storage.

Poultices. This is done by mashing the plant part (usually the leaves) with mortar and pestle and directly applying it to the affected area. This is good for external and local applications.

Chapter 5. Foods and Herbs That Have Antibacterial and Antiviral Properties

Taking antibiotic can kill bacteria within the body.

The problem with this statement is that it can kill bacteria in the body. Pharmaceutical antibiotics are able to kill bacteria but are unable to differentiate which is beneficial from which is not. More often than not, it kills both and causes more harm than benefits to the body as a result.

The complex antibacterial substances in herbs, however, are capable of killing specific strain of bacteria without harming the other. They also have almost zero side effects since they are natural and can strengthen the body and the immune system.

Among the many herbs that have antibacterial properties are:

Onions and garlic. Onions contain sulfur compounds that have antibacterial properties in addition to their anti-inflammatory properties. They are systemic and can be used both internally and external through local applications. In a study involving mice and a staphylococci superbug, it was found that the compound found in them (allicin and allistatin), enabled the rats to resist pathogens but reduced inflammation significantly as well. They are also known to have antifungal and antiviral properties. In addition, they high phytonutrients they contain can also help neutralize free radicals, which can lead to the formation of cancer in the body.

Honey. Known to have antibacterial properties, this sweet treat is known to be used as an antibacterial treatment long before antibiotics were formed. They are made with enzymes from the bees, which inhibit the growth of certain forms of bacteria and are used to disinfect wounds and neutralize toxins.

Fermented foods. Although they do not necessarily function as antibacterial, they are, on the other hand, good sources of probiotics. Probiotics are substances that encourage the growth of good bacteria in the intestines. In order to avoid the increase in the population of bad bacteria (and the associated illness), a certain degree of good bacteria population must be maintained. Fermented foods are rich in probiotics, which could encourage the growth of good bacteria, which competes in resources to, thereby limiting the population of, bad bacteria.

Marigold flowers. This non-systemic antibacterial is used to treat and facilitate the healing of wounds and prevent its infection. Since it is applied topically, it is prepared in either infusion, lotion, ointment and tincture forms. Prolonged use of the extracts of these Marigold flowers has been shown to have no side effects.

Cryptolepis. Also known by the names gangamau, kadze, Ghanaian quinine, yellow root and nibima, this plant has been used for years by the Ghanaian to treat malaria. The active compound in this herb able to kill Plasmodium falciparum and chloroquine-resistant variants are the indoquinoline, quindoline, cryptolepine and neocryptolepine alkaloids. The root of this plant, which is exceptionally bitter, is crushed and prepared into powder, tea, tincture or capsules. Cryptolepis is a systemic antibacterial herb and is absorbed into the bloodstream thereby effectively killing bacteria and Plasmodium. Researches and studies found that not observable adverse reactions both in the lab animals and in human trials. A compound taken from the roots of Cryptolepis called Cryptolepine is known to intercalate DNA—it inserts in between the double helix of the DNA and interfere with the cellular division of cancer cells. Because of the mechanism of action of this compound, it is known to have mild antiviral effects, too. It also acts as antiparasitic, antiprotozoal, antimalarial and anti-inflammatory agent.

Sida. This plant is among those few plants, which contain the cytotoxic and antimalarial compound Cryptolepine other than Cryptolepis and generate various derivatives such as quindoline, quindolinone and cryptolepinone. Similar to Cryptolepis, this plant is used to treat malaria and the associated symptoms such as fever and headache. It can also be used to treat various problems of the GI tract, systemic infections, diarrhea and infected wounds. This herb has been found to have no side effects.

Alchornea. This antibacterial and antiviral plant used to treat infectious diseases such as malaria, staph infections (even those that are resistant), diarrhea, dysentery and some resistant gram-negative and gram-positive infections. The parts used commonly are its fruits, roots, the bark of the root, the stem, the pith and the leaves.

Bidens. This systemic antibacterial and antiviral herb has a broad range of action as Cryptolepis or Sida although not as potent. It provides a reliable treatment, however, for various infections. It is used to treat, also, a number of resistant infections where conventional (or even the strongest versions) of pharmaceutical antibiotics no longer has effects. Studies about it have revealed that is has no potential side effects. However, it was found to produce alterations in the insulin and blood-glucose levels and must be introduced with caution to people suffering from diabetes and related diseases. In preparation, the entire plant can be used. Common preparation method used is tincture. Like the two anti-malarial herbs, Bidens is also regarded as one of the most active herbs against malaria. Studies also reveal that it can potentiate or increase the efficacy of tetracycline.

Artemisia. The active compound artemisin found in Artemisia is used to treat malaria, as well as infections cause by E. coli, Proteus vulgaris, Staphylococcus aureus, Salmonella typhi and Bacillus subtilis. Although extracts of the plant can be prepared with high concentration of artemisin, it can also be prepared through infusion. Artimisia also features antiviral properties as well. 1 in 4, though, reports side effects to Artimisia as mild nausea, vomiting, tinnitus, mild stomach pain and pruritus.

Berberine-containing plants. Berberine acts by interfering with how the bacteria stick to the mucous membrane though increased production of lipoteirchoic acid in bacteria. It is considered a non-systemic antibacterial herb, though, and can only be used for local applications. Berberine-containing plants include: American goldenseal, Mahonia, Berberis, Coptis, Phellodendron, Corydalis, Tinospora and Argemone. The plant parts used for local application are the bark, the bark of the roots, the leaves, resins, the roots and the stems. Common preparation methods include tincture and powder form. The powder from is applied directly to scrapes, cuts or even to the infected wound.

Juniper. This is a non-systemic antibacterial herb used for local applications. The parts used are the needles, berries, root, bark and wood. Common preparation methods are tincture, infusion and decoction. In tincture, it is advised that one must use 150 proof alcohol and use a part of plant part per five parts of solvent. The berries can be eaten, too, in order to relieve one of gastrointestinal discomforts. The powder form, on the other hand, is used to cure infected wounds.

Chapter 6. Role of Immune System

The human immune system is capable or curbing up bacterial activity. An important part of the herbal treatment is that there are herbs that could bolster the strength and functions of the immune system in addition to their antibacterial functions. Pharmaceutical antibiotics, however, work on the opposite way—it shuts the immune system down for its work to begin.

Along with using herbs to treat diseases, one must follow these simple steps in order to keep one's immune system at tiptop shape:

Eat fresh fruits and vegetables. The words that must be given emphasis, here are fresh, fruits, and vegetables. These foods are rich in antioxidants, which are capable of neutralizing free radicals (or superoxide toxins) and strengthening the immune system.

Supplement on Vitamin D. Studies reveal that during heightened immune activity, T cells scour the body for vitamin D in order to activate the body's natural immune response. Without this compound, the T cell is unable to perform the usual immune functions.

Exercise. Physical activity has been found to increase the body's natural T cell response and enhance the function of antibodies. Research reveals that those who engage even in minor exercise are less likely to suffer from simply infections.

De-stress. Stress is one of the many factors that weaken the immune system. One way of managing stress is by engaging in Yoga, praying, doing a hobby or keeping a journal.

Have enough sleep. Not having enough sleep equates to reduced T cells and proteins responsible for optimum immune function. A hormone melatonin is released during sleep. Insufficient sleep leads to low levels of this hormone and reduced immune system function. The ideal duration for sleep is 7-8 hours at night.

When herbs, both systemic and synergistic are taken in combination with a strong immune system, the ability of infectious bacteria to prosper is reduced. In this battle against nature's most notorious killers, we rely on two things: our body's own ability to resist infection and nature's provision for it. With these two powerful combinations, nothing can go against it.

Conclusion

What you just read are the secrets to harnessing nature's power to fight against the most deadly agents of this world. The tool to protect you against it and to rid your system of infection is now within your mind. It is now up to you to take action.

What you need to do next is provide yourself with the herbs by planting them within you area. This will give you easy and immediate access to those for preparation should you needs one. You also need to practice preparing them in various ways as this skill will enable you insight of how to change preparation parameters in the future to produce more potent and effective versions.

The information you just acquired should also be shared—not contained. You will realize, in the long run that having people who share the same information and interest greatly propel your endeavors forward.

May you be empowered to fight against the threat of deadly infectious diseases. May you be an agent against it.

Thank You Page

I want to personally thank you for reading my book. I hope you found information in this book useful and I would be very grateful if you could leave your honest review about this book. I certainly want to thank you in advance for doing this.

If you have the time, you can check my other books too.

Ingram Content Group UK Ltd.
Milton Keynes UK
UKHW021300050423
419696UK00020B/680